SLIMMING DOWN ON STEAK

A Carnivore Approach to Weight Loss.

BYRON FUNCK

Slimming Down on Steak: A Carnivore Approach to Weight Loss

Table Of Contents

Chapter 1: Introduction to the Carnivore Diet	3
Chapter 2: Getting Started	9
Chapter 3: Choosing the Right Meats	15
Chapter 4: Crafting Your Carnivore Meal Plan	21
Chapter 5: Cooking Techniques for Carnivores	27
Chapter 6: Managing Challenges	32
Chapter 7: Tracking Your Progress	38
Chapter 8: Long-Term Sustainability	44
Chapter 9: Success Stories	50
Chapter 10: Conclusion and Next Steps	56
More From This Author on Amazon Books	64
Thank You for Reading	66

Slimming Down on Steak: A Carnivore Approach to Weight Loss

Disclaimer

This book is for informational purposes only and is not intended as medical, nutritional, or professional advice. The contents are based on personal experiences, research, and general knowledge about the carnivore diet. Individual results may vary, and any significant dietary changes should be made in consultation with a qualified healthcare professional. The author and publisher disclaim any responsibility for any adverse effects or consequences resulting directly or indirectly from the use or application of the information presented in this book. Readers are encouraged to use their own judgment and seek professional guidance when necessary.

Chapter 1: Introduction to the Carnivore Diet

Understanding the Carnivore Diet

The Carnivore Diet is a dietary regimen that emphasizes the exclusive consumption of animal products, primarily meat, fish, and animal-derived foods. This approach starkly contrasts with conventional diets that advocate for a variety of food groups, including fruits, vegetables, grains, and legumes. Proponents of the Carnivore Diet argue that by eliminating carbohydrates and plant-based foods, individuals can achieve significant weight loss and improve overall health. The fundamental premise is that the human body is primarily designed to thrive on animal proteins and fats, which can lead to fat loss, muscle preservation, and enhanced metabolic function.

One of the key attractions of the Carnivore Diet for those seeking weight loss is its simplicity. The diet eliminates the need to count calories or track macronutrients, allowing individuals to focus solely on consuming animal products. This straightforward approach can reduce decision fatigue related to meal planning and can lead to more consistent eating habits. Moreover, many people report that they feel satiated after meals consisting of meat and animal fats, which can help curb cravings and reduce the urge to snack between meals, further supporting weight loss efforts.

Slimming Down on Steak: A Carnivore Approach to Weight Loss

The Carnivore Diet also has the potential to influence hormonal regulation in ways that may facilitate weight loss. By removing carbohydrates, the diet can lead to lower insulin levels, which is important as high insulin levels can promote fat storage. Additionally, the protein-rich nature of the diet can increase levels of hormones such as glucagon, which helps to mobilize fat stores for energy. This hormonal shift can create a favorable environment for weight loss, as the body adapts to using fat as its primary fuel source instead of carbohydrates.

While the Carnivore Diet may offer various benefits, it is essential to approach it with a clear understanding of the potential challenges. Nutritional deficiencies can arise from the exclusion of plant foods, particularly in vitamins and minerals that are abundant in fruits and vegetables. Therefore, individuals considering this diet should be mindful of their nutrient intake and may need to supplement certain vitamins, such as Vitamin C and fiber. Additionally, transitioning to a Carnivore Diet can lead to temporary digestive changes, including constipation or diarrhea, as the body adjusts to the high protein and low carbohydrate intake.

In conclusion, the Carnivore Diet presents a unique approach to weight loss, focusing exclusively on animal products that may help simplify dietary choices and enhance satiety. While many individuals have reported success in losing weight and improving health markers on this diet, it is crucial to consider the potential drawbacks and nutritional balance. As with any dietary change, consulting with healthcare professionals or nutritionists can provide personalized guidance to ensure that the Carnivore Diet is implemented safely and effectively, ultimately supporting individual weight loss goals.

The Science Behind Meat-Based Weight Loss

The science behind meat-based weight loss is rooted in the unique properties of animal protein and its effects on metabolism, satiety, and body composition. When individuals consume a diet rich in meat, they typically increase their protein intake significantly. Research indicates that protein is more thermogenic than carbohydrates or fats, meaning that the body expends more energy digesting and metabolizing protein. This elevated thermogenesis can contribute to a higher overall caloric expenditure, making it easier for individuals to create a calorie deficit necessary for weight loss.

Slimming Down on Steak: A Carnivore Approach to Weight Loss

In addition to boosting metabolism, protein from meat sources plays a crucial role in promoting feelings of fullness. High-protein diets have been shown to enhance satiety hormones, such as peptide YY and glucagon-like peptide-1, while suppressing hunger hormones like ghrelin. As a result, individuals following a meat-based diet often report reduced cravings and a lower overall appetite. This phenomenon can lead to a natural reduction in calorie intake without the need for strict calorie counting or portion control, making weight loss a more manageable and sustainable process.

Another important aspect of meat-based weight loss is its impact on body composition. Consuming adequate protein while in a calorie deficit helps to preserve lean muscle mass, which is often lost during weight loss efforts. Maintaining muscle mass is vital because muscle tissue burns more calories at rest compared to fat tissue. Therefore, a diet that emphasizes meat can help individuals maintain their metabolic rate during weight loss, leading to more effective fat loss and a reduced likelihood of regaining weight after the diet concludes.

Moreover, the carnivore diet's elimination of carbohydrate-rich foods can also play a role in weight loss. Reducing carbohydrates can lead to lower insulin levels, which not only promotes fat oxidation but also minimizes fat storage. Additionally, many individuals experience a reduction in water weight during the initial stages of a low-carb diet due to glycogen depletion, which can provide quick satisfaction and motivation as they see immediate results on the scale. This initial weight loss can boost adherence to the diet and encourage individuals to stick with their meat-based eating strategies.

Finally, a meat-based diet can be rich in essential nutrients that support overall health and well-being. Meat provides vital vitamins and minerals, such as B vitamins, iron, and zinc, which are crucial for energy metabolism and immune function. By focusing on nutrient-dense animal foods, individuals can ensure they are not only losing weight but also nourishing their bodies. This holistic approach to weight loss emphasizes that a diet rich in meat can be both effective and beneficial, making it a compelling option for those seeking to slim down while enjoying the taste and satisfaction of steak and other animal products.

Benefits of a Carnivore Diet

The carnivore diet, which emphasizes the consumption of animal products while excluding plant-based foods, has gained attention for its potential benefits in weight loss. One of the primary advantages is its ability to promote satiety. Animal proteins and fats are known to be more filling than carbohydrates, which can help reduce overall calorie intake. When individuals feel satisfied after meals, they are less likely to snack or overeat, making it easier to maintain a caloric deficit essential for weight loss.

Another significant benefit of the carnivore diet is its simplicity. By focusing solely on animal products, meal planning and preparation become straightforward. There are no complicated recipes or extensive grocery lists, which can often lead to confusion and poor dietary choices. This simplicity can be particularly advantageous for those who struggle with the complexities of traditional dieting methods. By eliminating the need to count calories or track macronutrients, individuals can more easily adhere to the diet over the long term.

Slimming Down on Steak: A Carnivore Approach to Weight Loss

The carnivore diet may also lead to improved metabolic health, which is crucial for effective weight loss. Some studies suggest that high-protein diets can increase the thermic effect of food, meaning the body burns more calories during digestion. Additionally, the absence of carbohydrates can help stabilize blood sugar levels, reducing insulin spikes that may contribute to fat storage. By fostering a more balanced metabolic state, the carnivore diet can enhance the body's ability to burn fat effectively.

Moreover, many people report experiencing increased energy levels and improved mental clarity when following a carnivore diet. This heightened state of alertness can help individuals engage in physical activities more effectively, further supporting weight loss efforts. Regular physical activity is vital for maintaining a healthy weight, and feeling energized can encourage consistent exercise routines. As individuals become more active, they may also find it easier to maintain their weight loss over time.

Lastly, the carnivore diet can lead to significant changes in body composition. Many practitioners of this diet report losing fat while preserving lean muscle mass, which is essential for overall health and a well-functioning metabolism. This shift can result in a more toned appearance, often motivating individuals to continue their weight loss journey. As they see these positive changes, it can create a reinforcing cycle of healthy habits that contribute to sustained weight management and overall well-being.

Chapter 2: Getting Started

Assessing Your Current Diet

Assessing your current diet is a crucial first step in embarking on a successful weight loss journey, especially when considering a carnivore approach. Understanding what you currently consume allows you to identify patterns, preferences, and areas for improvement. Start by keeping a detailed food diary for at least one week. Record everything you eat, including portion sizes and meal times. This exercise will help you gain a clearer picture of your daily caloric intake and macronutrient distribution, which is essential for making informed adjustments moving forward.

Next, evaluate the types of foods you consume. On a carnivore diet, you will be focusing primarily on animal products such as meats, fish, eggs, and select dairy. It's important to analyze your current consumption of these foods versus carbohydrates, sugars, and processed items. Take note of how often you indulge in non-carnivore foods and assess how they contribute to your overall diet. This reflection will not only highlight areas where you can eliminate unnecessary items but will also help you understand how these foods impact your energy levels and cravings.

Slimming Down on Steak: A Carnivore Approach to Weight Loss

Another important aspect to consider is your eating habits and routines. Are you eating mindfully or mindlessly? Do you tend to snack throughout the day, or do you have set meal times? Recognizing whether you eat out of hunger or boredom can provide valuable insights into your relationship with food. In the context of a carnivore diet, it may be beneficial to establish a structured eating schedule that emphasizes satiating, protein-rich meals. This can help you manage hunger and reduce the temptation to revert to carbohydrate-heavy snacks.

In addition to examining food choices and eating habits, it's essential to consider the emotional and psychological factors that influence your diet. Stress, anxiety, and emotional triggers can lead to unhealthy eating patterns, which may sabotage your weight loss efforts. Reflect on your emotional responses to food and identify situations where you may have turned to non-carnivore options for comfort. Acknowledging these triggers can empower you to develop healthier coping strategies, making the transition to a carnivore diet more sustainable and effective.

Finally, setting specific goals based on your assessment will provide direction for your weight loss journey. Determine what you want to achieve with the carnivore diet, whether it's losing a specific number of pounds, improving energy levels, or enhancing overall health. Use your initial assessment as a benchmark to measure progress. Regularly revisit your food diary and adjust your approach as necessary, ensuring that you remain committed to your goals while allowing flexibility for personal preferences. By thoroughly assessing your current diet, you will be well-equipped to embrace the carnivore lifestyle and achieve lasting weight loss success.

Setting Realistic Weight Loss Goals

Setting realistic weight loss goals is a crucial step in the journey toward achieving and maintaining a healthy weight, especially when following a carnivore diet. Unlike traditional diets that may emphasize calorie counting or food variety, the carnivore approach focuses on the consumption of animal products. This unique perspective necessitates a tailored approach to goal setting that aligns with the principles of the diet while also considering individual circumstances. By establishing achievable and specific goals, individuals can create a sustainable path to weight loss that encourages long-term success.

To begin with, it is important to understand that weight loss is not a linear process. Many factors influence how quickly or slowly one loses weight, including metabolic rate, physical activity level, and individual differences in body composition. Therefore, setting a goal of losing a specific number of pounds in a particular timeframe may lead to frustration if the desired results are not achieved as expected. Instead, a more effective strategy is to focus on incremental changes, such as aiming to lose one to two pounds per week. This approach allows for fluctuations and plateaus while keeping motivation high.

Slimming Down on Steak: A Carnivore Approach to Weight Loss

In the context of a carnivore diet, goals should also reflect the unique benefits of this eating strategy. For instance, rather than solely focusing on weight loss, individuals might consider setting goals related to improving energy levels, enhancing mental clarity, or experiencing fewer cravings. These holistic objectives can provide additional motivation and reinforce the positive health outcomes associated with a carnivore lifestyle. By broadening the scope of goals, individuals can celebrate progress that goes beyond the scale.

Tracking progress is another essential component of setting realistic weight loss goals. Keeping a journal or using an app to monitor food intake, exercise, and changes in body measurements can provide valuable insights into what works and what does not. This data can help individuals adjust their goals as needed, ensuring they remain relevant and achievable. Additionally, regular check-ins with a healthcare professional or nutritionist familiar with the carnivore diet can offer accountability and guidance, helping to keep goals aligned with personal health objectives.

Lastly, it is vital to practice self-compassion throughout the weight loss journey. Setting realistic goals means acknowledging that setbacks are a natural part of the process. Individuals may encounter challenges such as social situations, emotional eating, or changes in routine that can impact their ability to stick to their goals. By approaching these challenges with kindness and understanding, individuals can remain focused on their overall health and well-being rather than becoming discouraged by temporary obstacles. Embracing a mindset of resilience will ultimately support long-term success in achieving weight loss goals while following a carnivore diet.

Preparing for the Transition

Preparing for the transition to a carnivore diet requires a thoughtful approach to ensure a successful and sustainable shift. The first step is to educate yourself about the principles of the carnivore diet, which emphasizes the consumption of animal products while eliminating carbohydrates and plant-based foods. Understanding the benefits, such as weight loss, improved energy levels, and reduced inflammation, can provide motivation as you embark on this journey. Research various sources, including books, podcasts, and reputable websites, to gather insights and personal experiences from those who have successfully adopted this way of eating.

Next, it is essential to assess your current dietary habits and identify specific changes you need to make. Start by keeping a food diary for a week to track your intake and identify areas for improvement. This exercise will help you recognize your reliance on carbohydrates and processed foods. Once you have a clear picture of your current eating patterns, you can gradually begin to eliminate non-carnivore foods from your diet. This gradual approach can help mitigate withdrawal symptoms and make the transition less overwhelming.

Stocking your kitchen with suitable carnivore-friendly foods is another critical step in preparing for the transition. Focus on high-quality animal products, including various cuts of meat, organ meats, eggs, and dairy if tolerated. Consider sourcing your meat from local farms or butchers to ensure freshness and quality. Having these items readily available will simplify meal planning and reduce the temptation to revert to old eating habits. Additionally, familiarize yourself with cooking techniques that enhance the flavors of these ingredients, as this will make your meals more enjoyable and satisfying.

Slimming Down on Steak: A Carnivore Approach to Weight Loss

It is also important to prepare for potential challenges during the transition. Many individuals experience symptoms like fatigue, headaches, or digestive issues as their bodies adapt to a new way of eating. Being aware of these possibilities can help you mentally prepare for them. Consider joining online forums or local support groups where you can connect with others who are also transitioning to a carnivore diet. Sharing experiences and tips can provide encouragement and practical advice, making it easier to navigate any difficulties that arise.

Lastly, set realistic expectations for your weight loss journey on the carnivore diet. While many people experience rapid weight loss initially, it is crucial to focus on long-term sustainability rather than quick fixes. Establishing a routine that includes regular meal planning, mindful eating, and honest self-reflection on your progress will contribute to lasting success. Embrace the journey as an opportunity for personal growth, and remember that individual results may vary. Being patient and committed to your goals will ultimately lead to a healthier relationship with food and your body.

Chapter 3: Choosing the Right Meats

Types of Meat to Include

When embarking on a carnivore diet for weight loss, the types of meat you include are crucial for achieving your goals while ensuring nutritional balance. The primary focus should be on high-quality, nutrient-dense meats that provide essential vitamins and minerals. Red meats like beef and lamb are excellent choices, as they are rich in protein, iron, and B vitamins. These nutrients are vital for energy levels, muscle maintenance, and overall health, making them foundational components of a successful weight loss strategy.

In addition to red meats, poultry should also be a staple in your diet. Chicken and turkey are leaner options that can help reduce overall calorie intake while still providing ample protein. Skinless varieties are recommended, as they contain less fat. Incorporating a variety of poultry can help prevent dietary boredom and ensure a broader spectrum of nutrients. Consider incorporating different cooking methods such as grilling or roasting to enhance flavor without adding unnecessary calories.

Slimming Down on Steak: A Carnivore Approach to Weight Loss

Seafood is another essential category to include in a carnivore weight loss plan. Fish like salmon, mackerel, and sardines are not only rich in protein but also provide healthy omega-3 fatty acids, which are known for their anti-inflammatory properties and benefits for heart health. Shellfish, such as shrimp and scallops, are also low in calories and high in protein, making them an ideal choice for those looking to slim down. Including seafood in your meal rotation can diversify your nutrient intake and introduce a variety of flavors into your diet.

Organ meats, often overlooked, are another critical element of a carnivore diet. Liver, kidneys, and heart are packed with vitamins and minerals, including vitamin A, vitamin B12, and iron. These nutrient-dense options can significantly enhance your overall health and support weight loss by providing essential nutrients that may be lacking in muscle meat alone. While they may require some culinary experimentation, incorporating organ meats into your diet can yield substantial health benefits.

Finally, it is important to consider the quality of the meat you consume. Sourcing grass-fed, pasture-raised, and wild-caught options can greatly influence the nutrient profile of your meals. These types of meat typically contain higher levels of omega-3 fatty acids and are free from harmful additives and hormones. Prioritizing high-quality meats not only supports your weight loss efforts but also promotes overall well-being, making your carnivore diet both effective and sustainable in the long run.

Grass Fed vs Grain Fed

When it comes to choosing the type of beef that aligns with a carnivore diet for weight loss, the debate between grass-fed and grain-fed options is significant. Grass-fed beef comes from cattle that have been raised on a natural diet of grasses and forage, while grain-fed beef is derived from cattle that have been primarily fed grains, such as corn and soy. This dietary difference significantly impacts the nutritional profile of the meat, making it essential for those focused on weight loss to consider what they are consuming.

Grass-fed beef is often touted for its higher content of omega-3 fatty acids, which are beneficial for heart health and have anti-inflammatory properties. Additionally, grass-fed beef tends to be leaner than its grain-fed counterpart, providing fewer calories and less saturated fat. For individuals on a weight loss journey, the lower calorie density can be advantageous, allowing for larger portions without sacrificing dietary goals. This aspect may help maintain satiety while adhering to a calorie deficit, crucial for effective weight management.

Slimming Down on Steak: A Carnivore Approach to Weight Loss

In contrast, grain-fed beef generally offers a different set of nutritional benefits. It is typically higher in total fat, which can contribute to a richer flavor and a juicier texture. While this might be appealing to some, it is essential to recognize that the increased fat content can lead to higher calorie intake. For those focused on losing weight, grain-fed beef might not be the most suitable option, as it can be easier to consume excess calories without realizing it. Furthermore, the omega-6 fatty acid profile in grain-fed beef can be more pronounced, leading to an imbalance if consumed excessively.

Moreover, the environmental and ethical considerations surrounding beef production also play a role in this discussion. Grass-fed cattle are often raised on pasture, which can lead to better animal welfare conditions and a reduced environmental impact in terms of land use and carbon footprint. For individuals who prioritize sustainability in their dietary choices, opting for grass-fed beef can align with their values while also supporting a healthier lifestyle. By choosing grass-fed options, consumers can contribute to a more sustainable food system that promotes better health outcomes.

Ultimately, the choice between grass-fed and grain-fed beef will depend on individual preferences and dietary goals. For those committed to losing weight on a carnivore diet, grass-fed beef may provide a more favorable nutritional profile, promoting health benefits while aiding in weight management. Understanding the differences between these two types of beef enables individuals to make informed decisions that align with both their health objectives and personal values, ultimately supporting their journey toward a slimmer, healthier lifestyle.

The Importance of Quality

The importance of quality in the context of a carnivore diet cannot be overstated, especially for those focused on weight loss. When choosing meat and animal products, the quality of the food directly impacts not only the nutritional value but also the overall health benefits one can derive from the diet. High-quality meat, sourced from grass-fed, pasture-raised animals, provides essential nutrients like omega-3 fatty acids, vitamins, and minerals that are crucial for maintaining a healthy metabolism and promoting weight loss. In contrast, lower-quality options often contain additives, hormones, and unhealthy fats that can hinder progress and negatively affect overall health.

Quality meat also influences satiety, which is a key factor in any weight loss journey. When consuming higher-quality protein sources, individuals often experience increased feelings of fullness and satisfaction. This is largely due to the higher nutrient density found in better-quality meats. When the body receives adequate nutrition, it is less likely to crave additional food, leading to reduced caloric intake and more effective weight management. For those following a carnivore diet, prioritizing high-quality meats helps ensure that hunger is managed effectively, making adherence to the dietary plan easier.

Slimming Down on Steak: A Carnivore Approach to Weight Loss

Furthermore, the sourcing of quality meat often reflects the animal's diet and living conditions, which can affect the meat's flavor and texture. Grass-fed beef, for instance, tends to have a richer taste and tenderness compared to conventionally raised beef. Consumers who prioritize quality often report greater enjoyment in their meals, which can enhance the overall experience of following a carnivore diet. Enjoyment of food is an essential component of any sustainable weight loss strategy, as it fosters a positive relationship with food and reduces the likelihood of binge eating or cravings for less nutritious options.

In addition to physical satiety and flavor, the psychological aspect of consuming quality food should not be overlooked. Knowing that one is consuming ethically and sustainably sourced meat can foster a sense of well-being and satisfaction that contributes positively to mental health. This psychological boost can be particularly beneficial for those trying to lose weight, as it can lessen the emotional struggles often associated with dieting. A positive mindset is crucial in maintaining motivation and commitment to a weight loss plan, and quality food can play a significant role in nurturing this mindset.

Finally, investing in high-quality meat can also lead to long-term health benefits that extend beyond weight loss. A diet rich in nutrient-dense, high-quality animal products can promote better heart health, improved digestion, and enhanced overall wellness. These benefits are especially important for individuals on a weight loss journey, as they often face challenges related to energy levels and recovery. By emphasizing quality in dietary choices, individuals can not only achieve their weight loss goals but also lay the foundation for a healthier lifestyle that supports ongoing wellness.

Chapter 4: Crafting Your Carnivore Meal Plan

Sample Meal Plans

Sample meal plans can serve as a practical guide for those following a carnivore diet aimed at weight loss. The simplicity of the carnivore approach allows for a variety of meal options that prioritize animal-based foods while eliminating carbohydrates. Each meal plan can be tailored to individual preferences, but the core idea remains consistent: focus on high-quality protein and healthy fats to support weight loss and overall health.

Slimming Down on Steak: A Carnivore Approach to Weight Loss

A typical day on a carnivore diet might begin with breakfast options such as ribeye steak or bacon. Both are rich in essential nutrients and fats, providing lasting energy without the need for carbohydrates. Accompanying these protein sources with eggs can further enhance the meal's nutritional profile. Eggs are an excellent source of vitamins, minerals, and healthy fats, making them a staple in many carnivore meal plans. This combination not only fuels the body but also helps to keep hunger at bay until the next meal.

For lunch, consider a hearty serving of grilled chicken thighs or pork chops. These cuts of meat are flavorful and can be seasoned with herbs and spices to enhance taste without adding carbohydrates. Pairing the protein with bone broth can be beneficial, as it provides collagen and other nutrients that support joint health and digestion. This meal can be filling and satisfying, keeping energy levels stable throughout the afternoon and minimizing cravings for snacks.

Dinner can feature a prime cut of beef, such as a tender filet mignon or a juicy T-bone steak. These cuts are not only delicious but are also packed with iron and B vitamins, which are crucial for energy production. Complementing dinner with organ meats, like liver, can significantly boost nutrient intake and support overall health. A simple preparation method, such as searing or grilling, preserves the natural flavors of the meat, allowing for a satisfying end to the day.

Slimming Down on Steak: A Carnivore Approach to Weight Loss

Snacking on the carnivore diet can include options like beef jerky, pork rinds, or hard-boiled eggs. These snacks are high in protein and can be easily prepared in advance, making them convenient for those on the go. Staying hydrated is also essential, so incorporating bone broth or drinking plenty of water throughout the day is advisable. This meal plan not only emphasizes the variety within the carnivore diet but also underscores the importance of enjoying food while working towards weight loss goals.

Portion Control on a Carnivore Diet

Portion control is an essential aspect of any weight loss strategy, including the carnivore diet. While this diet primarily focuses on animal-based foods, managing portion sizes is crucial to achieving and maintaining a caloric deficit, which is fundamental for weight loss. The carnivore diet encourages the consumption of meat, fish, and animal-derived products, but without mindful portion control, individuals may inadvertently consume more calories than they need, hindering their weight loss efforts.

Understanding the macronutrient composition of the foods consumed on a carnivore diet is vital. Meat is rich in protein and fat, which can be satiating but also calorie-dense. Different cuts of meat have varying fat contents; for example, ribeye steaks are higher in fat compared to lean cuts like chicken breast or turkey. By being aware of these differences, individuals can make informed choices about their portions based on their specific dietary goals and caloric needs. This awareness can help prevent overconsumption, even when adhering strictly to animal-based foods.

Slimming Down on Steak: A Carnivore Approach to Weight Loss

Another important factor in portion control is recognizing hunger cues and differentiating between true hunger and emotional eating. Many people may find that, due to the high protein content of a carnivore diet, they feel fuller for longer periods. This satiety can lead to natural portion control, as the body may signal that it does not need additional food. However, it is essential to remain attuned to these signals and avoid eating out of habit or boredom. Practicing mindfulness during meals can help individuals listen to their bodies and make better decisions regarding portion sizes.

Meal planning can also significantly aid in portion control. By preparing meals in advance, individuals can allocate specific amounts of food for each meal, reducing the chances of overeating. Utilizing a food scale or measuring cups can assist in accurately assessing portion sizes, especially when trying new cuts of meat or recipes. This structured approach not only promotes portion control but also fosters a sense of discipline that can be beneficial for long-term weight loss success.

Lastly, it is important to remember that the carnivore diet is not just about restriction but also about nourishment. Ensuring that meals are balanced and include a variety of meats can provide essential nutrients while still adhering to portion control. Incorporating organ meats, for example, can enhance the nutritional profile of meals without leading to excessive calorie intake. By focusing on quality and mindfulness around portion sizes, individuals can successfully navigate the challenges of weight loss on a carnivore diet and achieve their health goals.

Snacks and Supplements

In the context of a carnivore diet, snacks and supplements play an essential role in maintaining energy levels and supporting weight loss goals. While the primary focus of this dietary approach is on whole animal foods, understanding how to effectively incorporate snacks can help manage hunger between meals and provide necessary nutrients. Choosing the right snacks can also prevent feelings of deprivation, making it easier to adhere to the diet long-term.

When considering snacks on a carnivore diet, options are often limited to animal-based foods. Jerky, pork rinds, and beef sticks are convenient choices that provide protein and healthy fats without the carbohydrates found in traditional snacks. These options are not only portable but also satisfy cravings while keeping you within the guidelines of the diet. Additionally, hard-boiled eggs can serve as a nutrient-dense snack, offering a good balance of protein and fat, and they are easy to prepare in advance.

Supplements may also play a significant role in a carnivore diet, particularly for individuals who are new to this way of eating or those who may have specific nutrient concerns. While a well-rounded carnivore diet can provide many essential nutrients, some individuals may benefit from supplementation, especially with vitamins A, D, E, and K, along with omega-3 fatty acids, particularly if their intake of fatty fish is limited. It's essential to assess personal health needs and consider consulting a healthcare professional before starting any supplement regimen.

Slimming Down on Steak: A Carnivore Approach to Weight Loss

Hydration is another crucial aspect to consider when snacking and supplementing on a carnivore diet. Staying well-hydrated supports overall health and can aid in weight loss by maintaining energy levels and promoting optimal digestion. Bone broth serves as an excellent option for both hydration and nutrient intake, as it is rich in electrolytes and collagen. Incorporating bone broth into your daily routine can help enhance your overall nutrient profile while keeping you satisfied.

Finally, portion control remains vital when choosing snacks and supplements. Even on a carnivore diet, it's easy to overindulge in calorie-dense foods, which can hinder weight loss progress. Keeping snacks portioned and being mindful of overall caloric intake will help maintain a calorie deficit necessary for weight loss. By focusing on nutrient-dense snacks, utilizing appropriate supplements, and ensuring proper hydration, individuals can effectively support their weight loss journey while enjoying the benefits of a carnivore diet.

Chapter 5: Cooking Techniques for Carnivores

Grilling and Roasting

Grilling and roasting are two of the most popular cooking methods that not only enhance the flavor of meat but also align perfectly with a carnivore diet focused on weight loss. Both techniques allow for the natural flavors of the meat to shine, minimizing the need for heavy sauces or added fats that can contribute unnecessary calories. When done correctly, grilling and roasting can produce tender, juicy cuts of steak that satisfy cravings while keeping calorie counts manageable.

Grilling involves cooking meat over direct heat, typically on a grill or barbecue. This method is ideal for cuts such as ribeye, sirloin, or flank steak, which can develop a flavorful crust while remaining juicy on the inside. To maximize flavor without adding calories, marinating the steak in simple seasonings like salt, pepper, and herbs can enhance its taste without compromising the carnivore approach. Cooking at high temperatures also helps to sear the meat, locking in moisture and creating a satisfying texture that can make a meal more enjoyable.

Slimming Down on Steak: A Carnivore Approach to Weight Loss

Roasting, on the other hand, is a dry heat cooking method that involves cooking meat in an oven. This technique is particularly beneficial for larger cuts of meat, such as a whole beef tenderloin or a prime rib roast. Roasting allows for even cooking and can produce a beautifully browned exterior while keeping the interior tender. Utilizing a meat thermometer can help ensure the steak reaches the desired level of doneness while preventing overcooking, which can lead to dryness—an undesirable quality in a weight loss-friendly meal.

Both grilling and roasting offer the advantage of cooking meat without the need for added oils or fats, allowing for a focus on the quality and flavor of the meat itself. Seasoning can be kept simple, relying on the natural taste of the beef. Incorporating herbs like rosemary or thyme can add aromatic flavors without impacting caloric intake. Additionally, these cooking methods allow for easy portion control, as it is simple to cut the cooked meat into appropriate serving sizes that fit within a weight loss plan.

Incorporating grilled and roasted meats into a carnivore diet can be both satisfying and effective for weight loss. By choosing lean cuts, paying attention to portion sizes, and using cooking methods that enhance flavor without adding calories, individuals can enjoy a variety of delicious meals. These techniques not only contribute to a sense of fullness and satisfaction but also support the overall goals of a carnivore diet, making it easier to stick to a weight loss journey while enjoying the rich flavors of quality beef.

Sous Vide Cooking

Sous vide cooking is a method that has gained significant popularity in recent years, especially among those following specific dietary approaches like the carnivore diet. This technique involves vacuum-sealing food in a bag and cooking it to a precise temperature in a water bath. The sous vide method ensures that food is cooked evenly, retains moisture, and enhances flavors without the need for added fats or oils, making it particularly appealing for those focused on weight loss.

One of the key benefits of sous vide cooking for carnivores is its ability to produce perfectly cooked meats. Traditional cooking methods often lead to overcooked or dry meat, which can be unappetizing and deter individuals from sticking to a healthy eating plan. With sous vide, you can set the desired temperature for your steak or other cuts of meat, allowing it to cook slowly and evenly. This results in a tender and juicy product that can enhance the enjoyment of meals while still adhering to a low-calorie diet.

Additionally, sous vide cooking allows for greater control over portion sizes and nutritional content. By measuring the amount of food you prepare and cooking it precisely, you can manage your intake more effectively. This is particularly beneficial for those on a carnivore diet, as it often involves consuming large quantities of meat. With sous vide, you can ensure that you are eating the right portion sizes necessary for your weight loss goals without sacrificing flavor or satisfaction.

Slimming Down on Steak: A Carnivore Approach to Weight Loss

Another advantage of sous vide cooking is its convenience. Once the food is sealed and placed in the water bath, it requires minimal attention, freeing you up to focus on other tasks. This aspect is particularly useful for individuals with busy lifestyles who may struggle to find time to prepare healthy meals. With sous vide, you can batch-cook your favorite cuts of meat, store them in the refrigerator, and simply reheat them as needed, ensuring that you always have a healthy option available.

Finally, sous vide cooking promotes a more thoughtful approach to food preparation and consumption. When you take the time to prepare and cook your meals using this method, you become more engaged with your food choices. This mindfulness can lead to better eating habits and a more profound appreciation for the quality of the ingredients you consume. For those on a carnivore diet seeking weight loss, adopting sous vide cooking can transform mealtime into a rewarding experience that aligns with both health goals and culinary enjoyment.

Quick and Easy Recipes

The carnivore diet, centered around animal products, offers a variety of quick and easy recipes that align with weight loss goals. These recipes emphasize high-quality meats while minimizing preparation time, making them suitable for busy individuals. By focusing on protein-rich foods, followers of this diet can enjoy satisfying meals that help curb hunger and promote weight loss without complicated cooking techniques.

Slimming Down on Steak: A Carnivore Approach to Weight Loss

One popular option is the classic steak and eggs breakfast. This dish can be prepared in under 15 minutes and provides a hearty start to the day. Simply sear a ribeye or sirloin steak in a hot skillet for a few minutes on each side to achieve the desired doneness. While the steak cooks, crack a couple of eggs into the same pan, allowing them to fry in the flavorful drippings. This combination not only delivers essential nutrients but also keeps you full longer, reducing the likelihood of snacking before lunch.

For lunch, consider a quick beef stir-fry. Begin by slicing thin strips of flank steak and sautéing them in a hot skillet with a bit of beef tallow or butter. Add some bone broth to the pan for added moisture and flavor, and let it simmer for a few minutes. This simple dish is packed with protein and can be customized with different seasonings to keep it exciting. Pair it with a side of crispy pork rinds for added crunch without the carbs, making it an ideal option for those on a carnivore diet.

Dinner can be equally effortless with a one-pan roasted chicken. Place bone-in, skin-on chicken thighs in a baking dish and season them with salt, pepper, and your choice of herbs. Roast in the oven at 400 degrees Fahrenheit for about 30-35 minutes until the skin is crispy and the meat is cooked through. This method allows for minimal cleanup while providing a delicious and nourishing meal. Serve the chicken with a side of homemade beef bone broth for a complete, satisfying dinner.

Snacks can also be quick and easy while adhering to the carnivore diet. Jerky/ Biltong made from grass-fed beef, is a great on-the-go option that can satisfy cravings between meals. Additionally, hard-boiled eggs are another convenient choice, providing protein and healthy fats. By preparing these snacks in advance, individuals can ensure they have satisfying options readily available, helping them stay on track with their weight loss journey while fully embracing the flavors and benefits of a carnivore lifestyle.

Chapter 6: Managing Challenges

Overcoming Cravings

Overcoming cravings is a crucial aspect of adhering to a carnivore diet, especially for those seeking weight loss. Cravings can often feel overwhelming and may trigger a return to old eating habits, which can hinder progress. Identifying the root causes of these cravings is the first step in developing effective strategies to combat them. Common triggers include emotional stress, environmental cues, and even habitual behaviors. By understanding these factors, individuals can begin to create an environment that supports their dietary goals.

Slimming Down on Steak: A Carnivore Approach to Weight Loss

One effective strategy to manage cravings is to ensure that meals are satisfying and nutrient-dense. The carnivore diet focuses on animal products, which provide high-quality protein and fats that can help maintain satiety. Including a variety of meats, such as beef, pork, lamb, and organ meats, can not only enhance taste but also ensure a wide range of nutrients that support overall health. When meals are fulfilling, the likelihood of experiencing cravings diminishes significantly. Prioritizing quality over quantity in food choices can transform how the body feels and reacts to hunger signals.

Another essential tactic for overcoming cravings is to stay hydrated. Often, what feels like a craving for food can actually be a sign of dehydration. Drinking water throughout the day can help manage these false cravings and keep the body functioning optimally. Additionally, incorporating electrolyte-rich foods, such as bone broth, can further support hydration and replenish essential minerals. Staying well-hydrated can mitigate feelings of hunger and make it easier to resist temptations.

Mindfulness techniques play a significant role in managing cravings. Practicing mindfulness involves being aware of the sensations and emotions that arise when cravings hit. This self-awareness allows individuals to differentiate between actual hunger and emotional or habitual urges to eat. Techniques such as deep breathing, meditation, or even short walks can provide a mental break and reduce the impulse to give in to cravings. By developing a more mindful approach to eating, individuals can cultivate a healthier relationship with food and reinforce their commitment to the carnivore diet.

Lastly, building a support system is vital in overcoming cravings. Engaging with communities, whether online or in-person, can provide encouragement and shared experiences that foster resilience against cravings. Sharing challenges and successes with like-minded individuals can offer accountability and motivation. Additionally, exploring resources such as meal plans, recipes, and cooking tips can enhance the carnivore diet experience, making it easier to stick to goals. By combining these strategies, individuals can effectively manage cravings and stay on track with their weight loss journey.

Dealing with Social Situations

Social situations can often present unique challenges for those following a carnivore diet, particularly when it comes to maintaining weight loss goals. Events such as parties, family gatherings, or dining out can create pressure to deviate from your dietary preferences. Understanding how to navigate these situations is crucial for sustaining your commitment to a carnivore lifestyle while still enjoying social interactions.

One effective strategy for managing social situations is to plan ahead. If you know you will be attending an event where food will be served, consider eating a satiating carnivore meal beforehand. This will help you feel full and less tempted by non-carnivore options. Additionally, you can bring your own dish, which not only ensures there is something compliant with your diet but also provides an opportunity to share your lifestyle with others. This proactive approach allows you to participate fully in the social experience while staying aligned with your dietary choices.

Slimming Down on Steak: A Carnivore Approach to Weight Loss

When dining out, it is beneficial to become familiar with the menus of restaurants you frequent. Many establishments offer options that can easily fit into a carnivore diet, such as steaks, burgers, or grilled meats. Do not hesitate to ask the staff for modifications, such as substituting sides with extra meat or requesting that sauces and dressings be omitted. Being assertive about your dietary needs can help create a more enjoyable dining experience without compromising your goals.

Social pressure can also arise from friends and family who may not understand or support your dietary choices. In these moments, it is important to communicate your reasons for following the carnivore diet clearly and confidently. Sharing your personal journey and the benefits you have experienced can foster understanding and respect. Additionally, consider inviting supportive friends or family members to join you in your carnivore meals, which can create a positive atmosphere and reduce feelings of isolation.

Lastly, maintaining a flexible mindset is essential when dealing with social situations. While it is important to stick to your dietary regimen, allowing for occasional deviations can be beneficial for your overall mental well-being. If you find yourself in a situation where you choose to indulge, do so mindfully and return to your carnivore practices immediately afterward. This balanced approach can help you enjoy life's social aspects while still prioritizing your health and weight loss goals.

Addressing Nutritional Concerns

Addressing nutritional concerns is crucial for anyone embarking on a carnivore diet, especially those focused on weight loss. While the premise of a diet primarily consisting of animal products can be appealing for its simplicity and direct approach to reducing body fat, it is essential to ensure that nutritional needs are fully met. This approach may raise questions about the adequacy of vitamins, minerals, and other essential nutrients that are typically found in plant-based foods. Understanding these aspects can help individuals navigate their dietary choices more effectively.

One common concern is the intake of vitamins and minerals, particularly vitamin C and fiber, which are abundant in fruits and vegetables. While it is true that animal products do not provide vitamin C in significant amounts, the body has mechanisms to adapt to lower levels of this vitamin. Additionally, certain cuts of meat, especially organ meats, can offer a wealth of nutrients, including B vitamins, zinc, and iron, which are crucial for energy metabolism and overall health. Including a variety of meats, such as liver and shellfish, can help bridge these nutritional gaps.

Another consideration is the balance of fatty acids in the diet. A carnivore diet can lead to an increased intake of saturated fats, which some studies suggest may impact heart health. However, it is important to differentiate between different types of fats. Many carnivore dieters find that incorporating fatty cuts of meat along with lean portions can provide a well-rounded intake of omega-3 and omega-6 fatty acids. Sources such as fatty fish can be particularly beneficial in maintaining a healthy balance of these essential fats while supporting weight loss efforts.

Slimming Down on Steak: A Carnivore Approach to Weight Loss

Hydration and electrolyte balance are also vital components of adhering to a carnivore diet. The shift to a meat-centric diet can lead to changes in fluid retention and electrolyte levels, especially sodium, potassium, and magnesium. Individuals may experience symptoms such as fatigue or muscle cramps if they do not adequately manage their electrolyte intake. Consuming bone broth and incorporating salt into meals can help prevent deficiencies and ensure optimal hydration, which is essential for maintaining energy levels and supporting weight loss.

Lastly, it is essential to listen to one's body and recognize the signs of nutritional deficiencies. While a carnivore diet can be effective for weight loss, it is not a one-size-fits-all approach. Regular check-ins on physical and mental health can help identify any issues that may arise from this dietary shift. Consulting with a healthcare professional or a registered dietitian who understands the carnivore diet can provide personalized guidance and support, ensuring that nutritional needs are met while achieving weight loss goals.

Chapter 7: Tracking Your Progress

Keeping a Food Journal

Keeping a food journal is a powerful tool in the journey of weight loss, especially for those following a carnivore diet. By meticulously tracking what you eat, you create a record that not only helps you stay accountable but also provides insight into your eating habits. This practice encourages mindfulness regarding food choices, portion sizes, and overall dietary patterns. For individuals adhering to a carnivore approach, this can be particularly beneficial as it allows for a clearer understanding of how different animal-based foods affect energy levels, satiety, and overall well-being.

When starting a food journal, it's crucial to include specific details about each meal. Document the type of meat consumed, along with any additional animal products such as eggs or dairy. Note the portion sizes, preparation methods, and any seasonings or sauces used. This level of detail can help identify which foods support your weight loss goals and which may not yield the desired results. For example, tracking how different cuts of meat or cooking methods influence your cravings or energy can refine your diet even further as you work towards your weight loss objectives.

Slimming Down on Steak: A Carnivore Approach to Weight Loss

In addition to meal details, recording how you feel before and after eating can enhance the value of your food journal. Emotional and physical responses to meals can provide critical feedback that might otherwise go unnoticed. For instance, you may find that certain meats leave you feeling fuller longer, while others may lead to cravings shortly after consumption. By analyzing these patterns, you can make informed decisions about your food choices, ensuring they align with your weight loss journey and overall health.

Another benefit of keeping a food journal is the capability to track progress over time. By reviewing your entries, you can identify trends in weight loss, energy levels, and overall satisfaction with your diet. This retrospective look can be incredibly motivating, as it highlights the successes and adjustments needed along the way. Additionally, a well-maintained journal serves as a reference point for troubleshooting any plateaus or challenges in your weight-loss journey, allowing for strategic modifications to your carnivore plan.

Lastly, sharing your food journal with a community, whether it be friends, family, or an online forum, can provide external motivation and support. Engaging with others who share similar dietary goals fosters accountability and can lead to valuable exchanges of tips and encouragement. The process of journaling, combined with community input, can enhance the effectiveness of your carnivore diet strategy, making it easier to stay committed to your weight loss goals while enjoying the benefits of a meat-centric lifestyle.

Measuring Weight Loss

Measuring weight loss effectively is crucial for anyone embarking on a journey to shed pounds, especially when following a specialized diet like the carnivore approach. Unlike traditional methods that may rely heavily on calorie counting or food tracking, the carnivore diet focuses on a select group of foods—primarily animal products. This necessitates a different strategy for tracking progress. Weight loss can be evaluated through various methods, including body weight, body measurements, and even subjective feelings of health and energy.

Firstly, tracking body weight remains the most common method for measuring weight loss. Regularly stepping on the scale can provide an immediate snapshot of progress. However, it's important to consider fluctuations due to factors such as water retention, muscle gain, or hormonal changes. For those on a carnivore diet, the initial stages often involve rapid weight loss, primarily due to water weight. As the body adapts to a lower carbohydrate intake, these fluctuations may stabilize, making it essential to focus on long-term trends rather than daily numbers.

Slimming Down on Steak: A Carnivore Approach to Weight Loss

In addition to weight, monitoring body measurements can provide a more comprehensive understanding of fat loss. Taking measurements of the waist, hips, thighs, and arms can reveal changes that the scale may not accurately reflect. Many individuals find that they lose inches even when the scale shows little to no movement. This is particularly relevant for those on a high-protein diet like the carnivore approach, as muscle mass may increase while fat decreases. Tracking these measurements regularly—ideally once a month—can serve as a motivating factor and offer a clearer picture of overall progress.

Another effective method for measuring weight loss is through the use of body composition analysis. This can involve techniques such as bioelectrical impedance analysis or skinfold measurements to assess fat versus lean mass. Understanding the composition of weight lost can provide insight into whether the body is losing fat, gaining muscle, or both. For those following a carnivore diet, where protein intake is elevated, a focus on muscle preservation and growth can lead to a healthier body composition, which is a more beneficial outcome than weight loss alone.

Finally, subjective measures such as energy levels, mood, and overall well-being should also be considered when assessing weight loss success. The carnivore diet can lead to significant changes in how individuals feel, both physically and mentally. As the body adapts to this way of eating, many report improvements in energy, clarity, and reduced cravings, which can be just as important as the numbers on a scale. By incorporating these various methods of measurement, individuals can create a well-rounded picture of their weight loss journey, ensuring they remain motivated and focused on their health goals.

Adjusting Your Diet as Needed

Adjusting your diet is an essential part of any weight loss journey, particularly when following a carnivore approach. As you progress, your body may respond differently to the foods you consume, necessitating tweaks to your meal plan. The key is to remain attuned to your body's signals and adjust your diet to ensure that you are meeting your nutritional needs while also promoting effective weight loss. With the carnivore diet focusing primarily on animal-based foods, understanding how to navigate these adjustments is crucial for long-term success.

Firstly, it is important to recognize that individual responses to dietary changes can vary widely. While some individuals may experience rapid weight loss at the outset, others may encounter plateaus or fluctuations. Monitoring your body's reactions through regular assessments can provide insights into how your current diet is affecting your weight loss efforts. Keeping a food journal can be beneficial, allowing you to track not only your food intake but also your energy levels, mood, and any physical changes. This information can help you identify patterns and determine if adjustments are needed.

When considering dietary adjustments, the quality of your food choices should be a priority. Even within the carnivore framework, there are variations in the types of animal products you can consume. Incorporating a variety of meats, organ meats, and animal fats can help ensure you are receiving a broad spectrum of nutrients. If you find that your weight loss has stalled, experiment with different cuts of meat or consider increasing your intake of organ meats, which are nutrient-dense and can provide essential vitamins and minerals that support overall health and metabolism.

Slimming Down on Steak: A Carnivore Approach to Weight Loss

Another crucial aspect of adjusting your diet is portion control. While the carnivore diet allows for a wide range of animal-based foods, it is still possible to overconsume. If you are not experiencing the desired weight loss, it may be beneficial to evaluate your portion sizes. Some individuals may find that smaller, more frequent meals help manage hunger and promote metabolic efficiency. Others may thrive on larger meals with extended fasting periods in between. Finding the right balance that works for you is essential in making sustainable dietary adjustments.

Lastly, be open to experimenting with your macronutrient ratios. The carnivore diet is predominantly high in protein and fat, but the proportion of each can be tweaked based on your personal goals and how your body reacts. If you feel sluggish or are not seeing the results you hoped for, consider adjusting the fat content of your meals or incorporating more lean proteins. Additionally, staying hydrated and including bone broth can support your overall health and enhance your weight loss efforts. Remember, the journey to weight loss is not linear, and adjusting your diet as needed will help you navigate the challenges and optimize your success on the carnivore diet.

Chapter 8: Long-Term Sustainability

Maintaining Weight Loss with the Carnivore Diet

Maintaining weight loss on the carnivore diet requires a strategic approach that focuses on the principles of this high-protein, low-carbohydrate lifestyle. The carnivore diet consists primarily of animal products, which can lead to significant weight loss due to reduced carbohydrate intake, increased satiety, and enhanced metabolic function. To sustain weight loss, it is essential to understand how to adapt and monitor your eating habits while ensuring that you meet your nutritional needs.

One of the key strategies for maintaining weight loss on the carnivore diet is to establish a consistent eating schedule. Regular meal times can help regulate hunger cues and prevent overeating. Many people find success with intermittent fasting, which can naturally reduce caloric intake while promoting fat oxidation. By limiting the eating window, individuals often consume fewer calories, making it easier to maintain a calorie deficit without feeling deprived. Tracking food intake can also be beneficial to ensure that you remain within your desired macronutrient ratios.

Slimming Down on Steak: A Carnivore Approach to Weight Loss

Another important aspect of sustaining weight loss is the quality of animal products consumed. While the carnivore diet allows for various meats, focusing on nutrient-dense options like grass-fed beef, wild-caught fish, and pasture-raised eggs is crucial. These foods provide not only protein but also essential vitamins and minerals that support overall health. Incorporating organ meats, which are rich in nutrients, can further enhance dietary variety and nutritional adequacy, making it easier to adhere to the diet long-term.

Physical activity plays a significant role in weight maintenance on the carnivore diet. Combining strength training with cardiovascular exercises can enhance muscle mass and metabolism, thereby supporting weight management efforts. Engaging in regular physical activity also provides psychological benefits, helping to reinforce the commitment to a healthy lifestyle. It can be particularly motivating to track progress in fitness alongside weight loss, creating a holistic approach to well-being.

Lastly, staying connected to a supportive community can greatly influence the ability to maintain weight loss on the carnivore diet. Joining online forums, social media groups, or local meetups can provide motivation, accountability, and valuable tips from others who share similar goals. Sharing experiences and challenges can foster a sense of belonging, making it easier to navigate the ups and downs of the weight maintenance journey. By leveraging community support, individuals can stay focused on their objectives and celebrate their successes together.

Incorporating Variety

Incorporating variety into your carnivore diet is essential for maintaining long-term adherence and ensuring you receive a balanced array of nutrients. While the carnivore approach emphasizes meat as the primary food source, it is crucial to diversify the types of meats and animal products you consume. Different cuts of meat and various animal products offer unique flavors, textures, and nutritional profiles. By including a range of meats such as beef, pork, lamb, poultry, and game, you can prevent meal fatigue and keep your dining experience enjoyable.

Consider the importance of varying cooking methods as well. Grilling, roasting, smoking, and slow cooking can transform the same cut of meat into entirely different dishes. For instance, a brisket can be smoked for a tender, flavorful experience, while a steak can be quickly seared for a different texture and taste. Experimenting with different preparations not only enhances the flavor but can also influence how satisfying and enjoyable your meals are, ultimately supporting your weight loss journey.

Incorporate organ meats into your diet as well, as they are nutrient-dense and often overlooked. Liver, heart, and kidneys are rich in vitamins and minerals that can complement the nutrients found in muscle meats. Including a variety of organ meats in your meals can help ensure you are not missing out on essential nutrients, particularly fat-soluble vitamins and minerals that are critical for overall health. This approach not only adds variety but also aligns perfectly with the principles of a carnivore diet.

Slimming Down on Steak: A Carnivore Approach to Weight Loss

Don't forget about the importance of sourcing high-quality meats. Grass-fed, pasture-raised, and ethically sourced meats tend to have better nutritional profiles and flavors than their conventional counterparts. By choosing a variety of high-quality meats, you enhance the overall quality of your diet while supporting sustainable farming practices. This can lead to a more satisfying and enriching eating experience, which is instrumental in maintaining motivation and commitment to your weight loss goals.

Finally, consider incorporating seasonal and regional varieties of meats into your diet. This not only supports local farmers but also encourages you to explore different flavors and textures that may not be available year-round. By embracing the diversity of meats available in your area, you can keep your meals exciting and varied, which is essential for sustaining your carnivore lifestyle. Ultimately, incorporating variety is not just about taste; it plays a critical role in ensuring your diet is well-rounded and enjoyable, making it easier to stick to your weight loss plan.

Transitioning to a Balanced Approach

Transitioning to a balanced approach within the framework of a carnivore diet is essential for sustainable weight loss and overall health. While the carnivore diet emphasizes meat consumption, integrating a balanced perspective can help individuals avoid potential pitfalls while maximizing the benefits. This transition involves understanding the importance of nutrient diversity, ensuring adequate hydration, and recognizing the role of lifestyle factors in weight management.

Slimming Down on Steak: A Carnivore Approach to Weight Loss

Incorporating a variety of animal-based foods can enhance nutrient intake while adhering to a carnivore diet. While red meat is often the primary focus, including organ meats, poultry, and fish can provide essential vitamins and minerals that may be lacking in a more narrowly defined diet. Organ meats, for example, are rich in nutrients such as vitamin A, B vitamins, and iron, which are crucial for energy levels and metabolic function. By diversifying the types of animal products consumed, individuals can support their weight loss goals while ensuring their bodies receive a comprehensive array of nutrients.

Hydration plays a crucial role in any weight loss plan, including a carnivore diet. Many individuals may overlook the importance of water intake, especially when consuming high-protein diets. Proper hydration can aid digestion, support metabolic processes, and help control hunger signals. It is important to drink adequate amounts of water throughout the day and consider electrolyte balance, particularly when transitioning to a diet lower in carbohydrates. Incorporating bone broth can be beneficial, as it not only contributes to fluid intake but also provides electrolytes and collagen that support joint and gut health.

Slimming Down on Steak: A Carnivore Approach to Weight Loss

While diet is a significant factor in weight loss, lifestyle habits also play a critical role in achieving long-term success. Prioritizing sleep, managing stress levels, and engaging in regular physical activity can enhance the effectiveness of a carnivore diet. Quality sleep helps regulate hormones that influence hunger and metabolism, while stress management techniques can prevent emotional eating and cravings for non-carnivore foods. Incorporating strength training or cardiovascular exercises into a routine can further support weight loss and improve overall body composition.

Ultimately, transitioning to a balanced approach while following a carnivore diet means recognizing that flexibility and moderation can enhance the experience. Rather than adhering strictly to a single food category, understanding the broader spectrum of animal-based nutrition and lifestyle factors can lead to more sustainable weight loss outcomes. Embracing a balanced mindset allows for the exploration of various food sources, leading to improved health, energy levels, and satisfaction with the diet. By fostering this balance, individuals can enjoy the benefits of the carnivore diet while achieving their weight loss goals effectively.

Chapter 9: Success Stories

Transformational Journeys

Transformational journeys in weight loss often encompass more than just changes in diet; they are profound shifts in mindset, lifestyle, and personal identity. For individuals embarking on a carnivore diet, these journeys can be particularly striking, as they challenge conventional dietary norms and promote a lifestyle centered around animal-based foods. This approach not only focuses on the reduction of carbohydrates but also emphasizes the importance of high-quality animal products, which can lead to significant changes in health, energy levels, and overall well-being.

One of the most notable aspects of the carnivore diet is its potential for rapid weight loss. Many individuals report shedding excess pounds quickly and efficiently, often due to the satiating nature of protein and fats. By eliminating carbohydrates, the body is encouraged to enter a state of ketosis, where it burns fat for fuel instead of glucose. This metabolic shift can lead to reduced hunger, making it easier for individuals to maintain a calorie deficit without feeling deprived. The simplicity of the diet allows for easier meal planning and reduces the temptation to snack on less nutritious options.

Slimming Down on Steak: A Carnivore Approach to Weight Loss

As participants navigate their transformational journeys, they often experience a variety of health benefits beyond weight loss. Many report improvements in mental clarity, mood stabilization, and increased energy levels. For individuals struggling with conditions such as insulin resistance, inflammation, or digestive issues, the carnivore diet can provide a level of relief that enhances their overall quality of life. As they witness these positive changes, individuals may find themselves more motivated to stick with the diet, reinforcing their commitment to a healthier lifestyle.

Support and community play crucial roles in these transformational journeys. Engaging with others who share similar goals and experiences can provide encouragement and accountability. Online forums, social media groups, and local meetups create spaces where individuals can share recipes, success stories, and challenges. This sense of belonging fosters a supportive environment that can help individuals stay focused on their objectives while also offering practical advice based on real-life experiences.

Ultimately, transformational journeys through the carnivore diet are about more than just physical changes. They encompass a holistic approach to health and wellness, encouraging individuals to redefine their relationship with food, their bodies, and their overall lifestyle. As they embrace this new way of eating, many find that their identities evolve alongside their bodies, leading to a renewed sense of purpose and fulfillment in their weight loss and health journey. By committing to this path, individuals not only aim for a slimmer physique but also seek a more vibrant and energized life.

Lessons Learned from Others

The journey of weight loss is often filled with challenges, and learning from the experiences of others can provide valuable insights. Many individuals have successfully navigated their weight loss journeys by adopting a carnivore diet, which emphasizes the consumption of animal products while eliminating carbohydrates. By examining their stories, we can uncover key lessons that can aid anyone looking to achieve their weight loss goals through this approach.

One significant lesson is the importance of meal planning and preparation. Many successful adherents of the carnivore diet emphasize the necessity of organizing meals ahead of time. This practice not only helps individuals avoid impulsive eating decisions but also ensures they have access to nutritious, satisfying options. By dedicating time to prepare meals in advance, one can maintain control over their dietary choices and make it easier to resist temptations that may arise in social situations or during busy days.

Slimming Down on Steak: A Carnivore Approach to Weight Loss

Another common theme among those who have embraced this diet is the importance of listening to one's body. Many individuals report that the carnivore diet leads to a heightened awareness of hunger cues and satiety signals. This feedback mechanism allows for more intuitive eating, which can be particularly beneficial in maintaining a healthy weight. By focusing on the body's natural responses and adjusting food intake accordingly, individuals can cultivate a sustainable eating pattern that supports long-term weight loss.

Community support plays a crucial role in the success of those following a carnivore diet. Many individuals find motivation and encouragement through online forums, social media groups, or local meetups. Sharing experiences, challenges, and successes with like-minded individuals fosters a sense of accountability and belonging. This camaraderie not only helps maintain motivation but also provides practical advice and tips that can make the transition to a carnivore diet smoother and more enjoyable.

Finally, it is essential to recognize the psychological aspects of weight loss. Many who have succeeded on the carnivore diet highlight the mental shifts that accompany their physical transformations. By focusing on the simplicity of a meat-based diet, individuals often experience a reduction in decision fatigue related to food choices. Additionally, celebrating small victories and setting realistic goals can build confidence and resilience. Understanding the psychological journey involved in weight loss can empower individuals to overcome obstacles and stay committed to their dietary changes.

Inspiring Tips for Your Journey

When embarking on a weight loss journey, especially one centered around the carnivore diet, it's essential to foster a mindset that embraces change and resilience. The first step is to set realistic and achievable goals. Instead of aiming for drastic weight loss in a short period, consider establishing smaller milestones. This approach allows for gradual progress, which can lead to sustainable results. Celebrate each achievement, no matter how minor, as this will help maintain motivation and positive reinforcement throughout your journey.

Meal planning is another vital aspect of the carnivore diet. Preparing your meals in advance can help eliminate the temptation to stray from your dietary goals. Focus on incorporating a variety of meats, including beef, pork, poultry, and fish, to keep your meals interesting and satisfying. Experimenting with different cooking methods, such as grilling, roasting, or slow cooking, can add diversity to your meals. Additionally, consider investing in high-quality cuts of meat. While they may be more expensive, the enhanced flavor and nutritional benefits can make the experience more enjoyable and fulfilling.

Slimming Down on Steak: A Carnivore Approach to Weight Loss

Staying hydrated is often overlooked but is crucial for overall health and weight loss. On a carnivore diet, you may not be consuming the same amount of water-rich foods as on other diets, so it's essential to drink plenty of water throughout the day. Consider adding electrolytes, especially sodium, potassium, and magnesium, to your routine, as these are vital for maintaining hydration and energy levels. Regularly monitoring your hydration status can help you feel more energized and focused, ultimately supporting your weight loss efforts.

Engaging with a supportive community can significantly enhance your journey. Whether through online forums, social media groups, or local meet-ups, connecting with others following a similar dietary path can provide motivation and accountability. Sharing experiences, recipes, and tips can foster a sense of belonging and encourage you to stay committed to your goals. Additionally, learning from others who have successfully navigated their weight loss journeys can offer valuable insights and strategies that you can incorporate into your own routine.

Lastly, it's important to practice patience and self-compassion. Weight loss is a journey that can have its ups and downs, and there will be times when progress seems slow or stagnant. Embrace the understanding that every individual's body responds differently to dietary changes, and fluctuations in weight are normal. Focus on the positive changes you are making in your health and lifestyle rather than solely the number on the scale. By cultivating a healthy relationship with food and your body, you can create a sustainable approach to weight loss that will benefit you long after you reach your goals.

Chapter 10: Conclusion and Next Steps

Recap of Key Takeaways

The carnivore diet emphasizes a high-protein, low-carbohydrate approach that can lead to effective weight loss. One of the key takeaways from this approach is the importance of prioritizing nutrient-dense animal products. These foods provide essential vitamins and minerals that support overall health while keeping hunger at bay. By focusing on quality cuts of meat, organ meats, and animal fats, individuals can enjoy satisfying meals that promote satiety and reduce the likelihood of overeating.

Slimming Down on Steak: A Carnivore Approach to Weight Loss

Another important aspect of the carnivore diet is its simplicity and ease of meal planning. Unlike traditional weight loss programs that often require calorie counting and complex meal prep, the carnivore approach allows for straightforward decision-making regarding food choices. This simplicity can reduce the stress often associated with dieting, making it easier for individuals to adhere to their nutritional goals. By eliminating non-carnivore foods, followers can streamline their grocery lists and meal prep routines, leading to greater consistency and success in weight loss efforts.

The carnivore diet also encourages a shift in mindset regarding food consumption. Many people struggle with cravings for sugary and processed foods, which can undermine weight loss attempts. By focusing solely on animal products, individuals can break free from the cycle of sugar addiction and learn to appreciate the flavors and textures of meat. This change in perspective can lead to a more sustainable relationship with food, as individuals become more in tune with their body's hunger cues and nutritional needs.

Additionally, the diet has been associated with various health benefits beyond weight loss. Many practitioners report improvements in energy levels, mental clarity, and digestive health. These positive effects can further motivate individuals to stick with the carnivore diet, reinforcing their commitment to their weight loss journey. Understanding that the benefits extend beyond just shedding pounds can create a more holistic approach to health and well-being.

Finally, community support plays a vital role in the success of those following the carnivore diet. Engaging with like-minded individuals can provide encouragement, share experiences, and offer practical tips for overcoming challenges. Whether through online forums, social media groups, or local meetups, connecting with others on a similar path can enhance accountability and foster a sense of belonging. This support network can be invaluable for maintaining motivation and celebrating milestones in the weight loss journey.

Encouragement for Your Weight Loss Journey

Embarking on a weight loss journey can be both exciting and daunting, especially when adopting a carnivore diet. This approach, which emphasizes animal-based foods, offers unique benefits that can support your weight loss goals. Understanding the principles of the carnivore diet and how they align with your objectives is crucial for maintaining motivation. Emphasizing protein-rich foods can help you feel fuller for longer, reducing cravings and the temptation to snack on less nutritious options. Remember that every meal is an opportunity to nourish your body and support your weight loss efforts.

Slimming Down on Steak: A Carnivore Approach to Weight Loss

To stay encouraged throughout your journey, focus on the progress you make rather than just the numbers on the scale. Many individuals experience fluctuations in weight due to various factors, including water retention and muscle gain. Instead of fixating solely on your weight, pay attention to how you feel, your energy levels, and your overall health. You may notice improvements in your mood, sleep quality, and physical performance, which can serve as powerful motivators. Keeping a journal to document these changes can help you recognize and celebrate your achievements, no matter how small they may seem.

Community support plays a vital role in any weight loss journey, and the carnivore diet is no exception. Engaging with others who share similar goals can provide inspiration and encouragement. Online forums, social media groups, and local meet-ups offer opportunities to connect with like-minded individuals who can share tips, recipes, and experiences. These connections can help you feel less isolated in your journey, reminding you that you are not alone in your struggles and triumphs. Sharing your successes with others can boost your confidence and commitment to the diet.

Slimming Down on Steak: A Carnivore Approach to Weight Loss

It's important to have realistic expectations as you navigate your weight loss journey on a carnivore diet. While quick fixes and rapid results are enticing, sustainable weight loss often takes time and consistent effort. Embrace the idea that this is a lifestyle change rather than a temporary diet. Set achievable milestones and recognize that plateaus are a normal part of the process. By maintaining a long-term perspective, you can cultivate patience and resilience, which are essential for lasting success.

Finally, remember to be kind to yourself throughout this journey. Weight loss is not a linear process, and setbacks are likely to occur. Instead of viewing these moments as failures, consider them opportunities for learning and growth. Celebrate your commitment to the carnivore diet and the healthier choices you make every day. Each step forward, no matter how small, is a step toward your ultimate goal. By fostering a positive mindset and embracing the journey, you can create a fulfilling experience that leads to lasting weight loss and improved well-being.

Resources for Further Learning

For those looking to delve deeper into the carnivore diet and its implications for weight loss, a variety of resources are available that can enhance understanding and effectiveness. Numerous books have been published that detail the principles of the carnivore diet, its benefits, and how it can be integrated into a weight loss regimen. Titles such as "**The Carnivore Diet**" by **Shawn Baker** and "Meat Heals" by Kelly Hogan provide firsthand accounts and scientific insights that can help readers navigate their journey. These texts often include meal plans, recipes, and personal testimonials that illustrate the diet's potential for weight loss and overall health improvement.

In addition to traditional literature, online platforms offer a wealth of information on the carnivore diet. Websites dedicated to low-carb and carnivore lifestyles, such as MeatRx and Carnivore Diet Coach, serve as hubs for resources, including forums, articles, and expert advice. These platforms enable individuals to connect with others who share similar goals, fostering a community of support that can be invaluable during the weight loss journey. Engaging with these online communities allows for the exchange of tips, recipes, and encouragement, making the process more enjoyable and effective.

Slimming Down on Steak: A Carnivore Approach to Weight Loss

Podcasts and YouTube channels focused on the carnivore diet also provide dynamic resources for further learning. Many experts in the field share their insights, interview prominent figures, and discuss emerging research related to meat-based diets and weight loss. Shows like "The Carnivore Cast" and *YouTube channels* such as "**Dr. Anthony Chaffee**" explore various aspects of the diet, including its impact on metabolism, energy levels, and mental clarity. These auditory and visual resources can be particularly helpful for those who prefer learning through listening or watching rather than reading.

Social media platforms, particularly Instagram and Facebook, have become popular venues for sharing information and success stories related to the carnivore diet. Influencers and health coaches often post meal ideas, tips for staying motivated, and personal experiences that resonate with followers. Engaging with these accounts can provide inspiration and practical advice, making the transition to a carnivore diet less daunting. Following hashtags like **#CarnivoreDiet** or **#MeatBasedDiet** can lead to a treasure trove of user-generated content that showcases diverse approaches to weight loss through carnivorous eating.

Slimming Down on Steak: A Carnivore Approach to Weight Loss

Finally, professional guidance is an essential resource for those serious about adopting the carnivore diet for weight loss. Consulting with a registered dietitian or nutritionist who specializes in low-carb or carnivore diets can provide personalized advice tailored to individual health needs and goals. These professionals can help create a balanced approach that ensures nutritional adequacy while promoting weight loss. Whether through one-on-one sessions, workshops, or group classes, professional support can significantly enhance the effectiveness of the carnivore diet and address any concerns that may arise during the journey.

More From This Author on Amazon Books

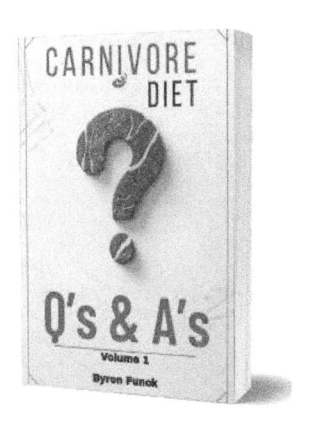

Carnivore Diet Q's & A's Vol. 1
Click here to explore!

V1: Straightforward answers to common carnivore diet questions. Whether you're just starting or looking for clarity, this book provides science-backed insights and practical tips to help you succeed on a meat-based diet.

Slimming Down on Steak: A Carnivore Approach to Weight Loss

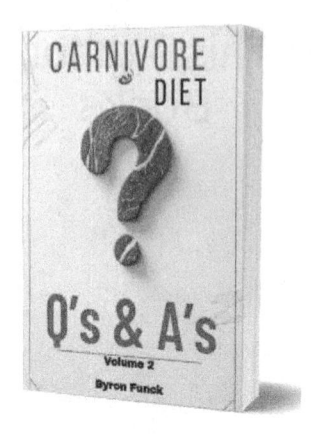

Carnivore Diet Q's & A's Vol. 2
Click here to explore!

V2: Diving deeper into the carnivore lifestyle, this second volume tackles the most pressing and controversial questions about long-term health, nutrient optimization, and troubleshooting common challenges.

Thank You for Reading

I hope you found Slimming Down on Steak helpful on your journey to better health and weight loss. If this book provided value to you, I'd truly appreciate it if you could leave a quick review on Amazon. Your feedback helps others discover this book and supports future content creation.

Share with a Friend!
Know someone interested in the carnivore diet? Share this book with them and help them get started on their journey!

Want More Carnivore Insights? Check out my Carnivore Diet Q's & A's series for even more answers to your burning questions!

Carnivore Diet Q's & A's Vol. 1
Carnivore Diet Q's & A's Vol. 2

Thank you for your support!
Stay strong and keep thriving on your carnivore journey.

Burn Fat. Boost Energy. Simplify Your Diet. Struggling with weight loss? Slimming Down on Steak reveals how a meat-based diet can help you shed fat, gain energy, and transform your health—without counting calories or complicated meal plans. The science behind carnivore weight loss Easy meal plans & cooking techniques How to overcome cravings & stay on track Success stories & expert-backed insights Take control of your health. Start your carnivore journey today!

Made in the USA
Las Vegas, NV
28 March 2025